AMD

AGE-RELATED MACULAR

DEGENERATION

AMD

AGE-RELATED MACULAR
DEGENERATION

Dr. Jean-Daniel Arbour, Dr. Francine Behar-Cohen,
Dr. Pierre Labelle and Dr. Florian Sennlaub

Preface by Dr. Alan F. Cruess

AP Annika Parance Publishing

*Bibliothèque et Archives nationales du Québec and
Library and Archives Canada cataloguing in publication*

Main entry under title:

AMD, age-related macular degeneration: understanding AMD and its treatment

Translation of: DMLA, la dégénérescence maculaire liée à l'âge.
Includes bibliographical references.
ISBN 978-2-923830-01-8

1. Retinal degeneration - Popular works. 2. Retinal degeneration - Treatment - Popular works. I. Arbour, Jean-Daniel, 1964- .

RE661.D3D5413 2010   617.7'35   C2010-940662-1

Annika Parance Publishing
4067 St. Lawrence Blvd.
Suite 400
Montreal, Quebec
H2W 1Y7
514-658-7217

Contributing editor: Frédérique David
Translation: Debby Dubrofsky
Book and cover design: Francis Desrosiers in collaboration with Scalpel design

Photographs and diagrams reproduced with permission from Novartis Pharma Canada Inc. and the Institut Nazareth & Louis-Braille.

Legal deposit – Bibliothèque et Archives nationales du Québec, 2010
Legal deposit – Library and Archives Canada, 2010

This publication is made possible through an unrestricted educational grant from Novartis Pharma Canada inc. and the Antoine-Turmel Foundation.

Printed in Canada

CONTENTS

CHAPTER 2
THE TWO FORMS OF AMD   35

CHAPTER 3
RISK FACTORS   51

CHAPTER 4
DIAGNOSIS 61

CHAPTER 5
PREVENTION AND TREATMENT 75

CHAPTER 7
TREATMENTS OF THE FUTURE 105

THE AUTHORS

Dr. Jean-Daniel Arbour
Dr. Jean Daniel Arbour heads the ophthalmology department of the faculty of medicine at the University of Montreal, where he is also associate professor.

After receiving his M.D. from the University of Montreal, Dr. Arbour interned in general surgery, specialized in ophthalmology and then went to Harvard University in the United States for medical and surgical retina training. At Harvard, Dr. Arbour also conducted research on macular degeneration and photodynamic and antiangiogenic therapy.

Dr. Arbour is currently vitreoretinal surgeon at Notre-Dame Hospital, which is part of the University of Montreal hospital centre (CHUM). He is also the founder of the hospital's ophthalmology research centre, where he has been the principal investigator in genetic studies of wet AMD and numerous international studies of new treatments in macular degeneration and diabetic retinopathy. The author of many articles published in medical journals, Dr. Arbour has also given more than 70 national and international scientific conferences on retinal disease.

Dr. Arbour was president of the Quebec association of ophthalmologists from 2005 to 2009. He is currently treasurer of the Canadian Ophthalmological Society.

Dr. Francine Behar-Cohen

Dr. Francine Behar-Cohen has served as professor and staff ophthalmologist at the Hôtel-Dieu de Paris since 2006. A retinologist, she is currently setting up a clinical research unit. Dr. Behar-Cohen received her M.D. and a Ph.D. in cellular biology from the Paris-Descartes University and did her internship in Paris hospitals and her residency in vitreoretinal surgery at the Hôtel-Dieu de Paris.

In 2001, Dr. Behar-Cohen headed an Avenir team at France's national institute of health and medical research (INSERM,) and in 2003 she founded INSERM Unit 598, dedicated to the physiopathology of eye diseases and therapeutic innovations. In 2008, this unit became the Cordelier Research Center, located in Paris.

Dr. Behar-Cohen has been researching ocular drug delivery systems and pharmacology for more than ten years. She is also investigating intraocular inflammation and the role of inflammation in retinal pathologies previously considered noninflammatory—including ADM and diabetic retinopathy. She is the author of more than 110 publications and about a dozen books or book chapters.

Dr. Pierre Labelle

Dr. Pierre Labelle is an ophthalmologist at Maisonneuve-Rosemont Hospital and full clinical professor in the department of ophthalmology of the faculty of medicine at the University of Montreal.

After receiving his M.D. and his diploma in ophthalmology, Dr. Labelle completed a research fellowship in retinal diseases and surgery at Washington University in St. Louis in the United States. He earned the first medal awarded by the Canadian Ophthalmological Society for his work on the prevention of sports-related eye injuries and was awarded the Securitas prize by the *Régie de la sécurité dans les sports du Québec*, Quebec's sports safety board, for his public awareness work.

Dr. Labelle is president of the *Association des médecins ophtalmologistes du Québec*, Quebec's association of ophthalmologists, and heads the ophthalmology departments of Maisonneuve-Rosemont Hospital and the faculty of medicine of the University of Montreal. Under his direction, the Centre Michel-Mathieu was established at Maisonneuve-Rosemont Hospital in 1999, an internationally renowned institute of excellence in ophthalmology. Given his interest in clinical research, Dr. Labelle has collaborated on many research projects, including projects investigating macular degeneration.

Dr. Florian Sennlaub

Dr. Florian Sennlaub heads a research team at France's national institute of health and medical research (INSERM) in Paris. Born in Germany, Dr. Sennlaub studied medicine in Germany, Scotland and France. He received his M.D. from the University of Humboldt in Berlin and a Ph.D. from René-Descartes University in Paris before devoting himself full-time to research in ophthalmology.

He worked for three years at the research centre at Sainte-Justine Hospital in Montreal before putting together his own team to explore the mechanisms of ocular degeneration and neovascularization at the Cordelier Research Center in Paris. Dr. Sennlaub regularly publishes articles in journals specializing in biomedical research. His research is supported by French and European agencies.

SPECIAL CONTRIBUTOR TO CHAPTER 6, LIVING WITH AMD

Julie-Andrée Marinier

Optometrist and assistant professor at the school of optometry at the University of Montreal, Julie-Andrée Marinier also serves as low-vision optometrist at the Institut Nazareth et Louis-Braille (INLB) in Montreal.

She received her Doctor of Optometry degree and an M.Sc. in Vision Science from the University of Montreal. Her M.Sc. dissertation, completed in 2003, examines the investigation of choroidal blood flow in AMD. She has also contributed to numerous articles in medical journals and given conferences on AMD.

PREFACE

Age-related macular degeneration (AMD) is the leading cause of visual loss in people over the age of 65.[1,2] It is a chronic, progressive, neurodegenerative disease of the retina and choroid resulting in central visual loss (including loss of reading and driving abilities), a very significant loss in quality of life and a high burden of illness for society. There are an estimated 25 to 30 million people worldwide with AMD,[3] and the number is expected to double by 2020.

General understanding of AMD among the public has been limited, in part because of the lack of therapeutic options for the exudative or neovascular form of the disease prior to the advent of photodynamic therapy and anti-vascular endothelial growth factor (anti-VEGF) treatment. AMD occurs in two forms: the more common dry or atrophic form; and the less common wet or exudative form associated with choroidal neovascularization, which causes a more rapid and devastating visual loss.

Recent treatment advances have all involved anti-VEGF therapies directed towards the wet form of the disease to curb and induce involution of the underlying choroidal neovascularization—which leads to scarring in the macular retina if left unchecked. While there is no active therapy to halt or reverse the progression of the dry or atrophic form of the disease, healthy lifestyle choices, including smoking cessation and a healthy diet rich in anti-oxidants, zinc-containing foods and omega-3 fatty acids (found in fish) can slow the progression of disease.

Recently, major advances have been made in our understanding of the biology of macular degeneration and the genetic basis of the disease, throwing light on the possible role of inflammatory processes (involving complement and other proteins) and programmed cell death or apoptosis in the pathophysiology of the disease, in both its dry and wet forms. This new knowledge in turn is driving new research into potential drug targets along the cascade of biological events that lead to visual loss in AMD. We thus have reason to expect exciting new treatment and prevention options in the near future.

This book by professors Jean-Daniel Arbour, Francine Behar-Cohen, Pierre Labelle and Florian Sennlaub makes a very important contribution to improving our understanding of this major cause of visual disability. A better-informed public will result in better questions being asked of caregivers, eye-care professionals, ophthalmologists and governments responsible for policy-making in vision care—all of which will lead to improvements in quality of and access to timely care.

The strategic application of public funding to improve access to and funding for innovative treatments and vision rehabilitation services and to reduce the burden of this major cause of visual loss must be given the highest priority.

Alan F. Cruess, MD, FRCSC
Professor and Head
District Chief, Capital Health
Department of Ophthalmology and Visual Sciences
Dalhousie University, Halifax, Nova Scotia

References
1. Ambati J, Ambati BK, Yoo SH, Lanchulev S, Adamis AP. Age-related macular degeneration: etiology, pathogenesis, and therapeutic strategies. *Surv Ophthalmol* 2003;48(3):257-93.
2. Vingerling JR, Klaver CC, Hofman A, de Jong PT. Epidemiology of age-related maculopathy. *Epidemiol Rev* 1995;17(2):347-59.
3. Verma L, Das T, Binder S, *et al.* New approaches in the management of choroidal neovascular membrane in age-related macular degeneration. *Indian J Ophthalmol* 2000;48:263-78.

25 FREQUENTLY ASKED QUESTIONS

(1) Is AMD a common disorder?

About 25 to 30 million people worldwide are affected by AMD, including one million in Canada. AMD is the leading cause of severe vision loss in people over the age of 55 in the industrialized world. The dry form accounts for 85 to 90 percent of AMD patients, and the wet form for 10 to 15 percent. Overall prevalence of AMD increases gradually with age: it affects about one to two percent of people between 50 and 65 years of age, 10 percent between 65 and 75 years of age and 25 percent between 75 and 85 (Chapter 1).

② What are the symptoms of AMD?

The most common symptoms of AMD are a need for more light when reading, a gradual reduction in far and near visual acuity and sometimes distortion of straight lines (metamorphopsia) and appearance of dark or blurry areas (scotoma). Changes in vision may not be noticeable at the beginning (Chapter 2).

③ What are the causes of AMD?

No one knows exactly what causes AMD. Probably there are a number of factors involved. We do know, however, that age and family history are two major risk factors (Chapter 3).

④ Does AMD cause blindness?

AMD does not cause blindness. It causes a loss of both near and far central vision, which can make certain activities, such as reading, difficult. Peripheral vision remains intact, which means those affected can get around on their own (Chapter 1).

⑤ How do you know you have AMD?

An optometrist or ophthalmologist can detect AMD by examining the back of the eye (ocular fundus examination), which will also indicate the type and severity of the disease (Chapter 4).

⑥ When is an emergency visit required?

An emergency consultation with a vision specialist is required when a sudden major change in vision is noticed (Chapter 4).

⑦ Is AMD caused by overusing the eyes?

AMD is not caused by prolonged reading, working at a computer, watching television or intensive use of the eyes for close work (Chapter 3).

⑧ Can AMD be triggered by certain drugs?

To date, the onset of AMD has not been associated with use of any medication (Chapter 4).

⑨ Can AMD be prevented?

There is currently no known preventive therapy for AMD. However, an antioxidant-rich diet may protect against AMD (Chapter 5).

⑩ Is AMD hereditary?

Recent data suggest AMD is hereditary in some cases. Scientists have recently identified some of the genes associated with macular degeneration (Chapter 5).

⑪ Can AMD be cured?

There is no treatment for the dry form of AMD, but its progression can sometimes be slowed by taking nutritional supplements. The wet form of AMD, which is more rare but also more aggressive, can be stopped. Available treatments can often lead to an improvement in vision (Chapter 5).

⑫ Can the progression of AMD be slowed?

Yes. Existing therapies have proven effective in slowing the progression of symptoms of AMD. Even better, certain treatments for the wet form can improve vision (Chapter 5).

⑬ Can an operation be performed?

There is no operation that can cure AMD. Surgery is used in AMD only in rare cases of massive hemorrhage (see Chapter 5).

⑭ If one eye is affected, will the other be automatically affected?

Signs and symptoms of AMD may appear in only one eye at first. Eventually, both eyes will be affected, though severity and speed of vision loss will differ. Close to 50 percent of people with wet AMD in one eye will be affected in both eyes within five years (Chapter 2).

⑮ How often should a specialist be consulted?

Monitoring by an optometrist or an ophthalmologist is indispensable if you have AMD. The treatment required and the frequency of visits will be determined by your vision specialist (Chapter 5).

⑯ Is AMD painful?

No, AMD is not painful. The eye examinations required and the treatments available are not painful either (Chapter 2).

⑰ Can you drive if you have AMD?

Most people with AMD keep their driver's licenses for a very long time. Corrected visual acuity must be not less than 6/15 (20/50) to drive in Canada. When AMD causes a major loss of visual acuity, the patient is no longer able to drive (Chapter 6).

Can you take a plane if you have AMD?

Yes. Air pressure changes in an airplane do not pose a risk for people with AMD (Chapter 6).

 Can you live alone if you have AMD?

Most people with AMD can continue to live alone without difficulty. However, the person's physical condition and the layout of the home (stairs, etc.) are important factors (Chapter 6).

 Can you get around on your own if you have AMD?

Yes. Certain tools have been developed to make it easier for people who are visually impaired to get around— tactile transit system maps, for example (Chapter 6).

㉑ **Are there vision aids that can help?**

There are numerous vision aids (magnifiers, closed circuit televisions, etc.) that facilitate daily activities for people with AMD (Chapter 6).

㉒ **Can vision loss due to AMD be recovered by a change of glasses?**

No, glasses cannot bring back vision lost. No matter what type of glasses are used, the dark spot will always remain in the field of vision of people with AMD (Chapter 6).

㉓ **Should people with AMD change their diet?**

A very well-balanced diet and certain food guidelines are recommended for people with AMD: lots of fruits, vegetables and fish, and little fat (chapters 3 and 5).

㉔ Should people with AMD quit smoking?

It's always a good idea to quit smoking. Smokers are at higher risk of developing AMD. Recent studies also show that people with AMD who continue to smoke increase their risk of developing a more severe form of the disease (chapters 3 and 5).

㉕ Should people with AMD take nutritional supplements?

An ophthalmologist may prescribe nutritional supplements (antioxidants) for anyone with dry AMD at high risk of developing wet AMD. However, nutritional supplements cannot substitute for a healthy, varied and balanced diet (Chapter 5).

CHAPTER 1
UNDERSTANDING AMD

Age-related macular degeneration (AMD) affects 12 percent of the population between 65 and 75 years of age in the Western world,[1] including an estimated one million Canadians.[2] A chronic, degenerative disease, AMD is the leading cause of severe vision loss after age 55 in industrialized countries.[3] However, the public is still relatively unfamiliar with AMD, despite its high incidence. With our aging populations, the number of people with AMD may increase by close to 50 percent by 2020.[4] A major public health issue, AMD has been the subject of much research, and important progress has been made.

WHAT IS AMD?

AMD is caused by progressive degeneration (premature aging) of the macula. White deposits, called drusen, appear in the central part of the retina, and cells (photoreceptors and pigment epithelial cells) disappear, causing a gradual loss of near and far central vision. There are two forms of AMD, the dry form and the wet form (*see Chapter 2*). Generally, peripheral or lateral vision remains intact. This disease of the retina usually occurs after age 50 and mainly after age 65. It causes major visual impairment but does not lead to blindness.

AMD is twice as prevalent among Caucasians as among black people, while Asians and Hispanics fall somewhere between.

Let's take a closer look now at how the eye works, the retina in particular, to get a better understanding of how AMD affects vision.

HOW THE EYE AND THE RETINA WORK

The eye is a spherical organ about 2.5 centimetres (one inch) in diameter consisting of several covering layers plus internal structures (*Figure* ❶). Only part of the eye is visible; the rest is hidden inside the skull. The eye is often said to work like a 35-mm camera (before the advent of digital cameras): to get a clear, crisp image, we adjust the focus and then the diaphragm opens and closes to let in the right amount of light. The same principle applies to the eye. The image is focused by the cornea and the lens, and the iris serves as the diaphragm. The image thus formed is projected onto the retina, which lines the back of the eye like film in a camera.

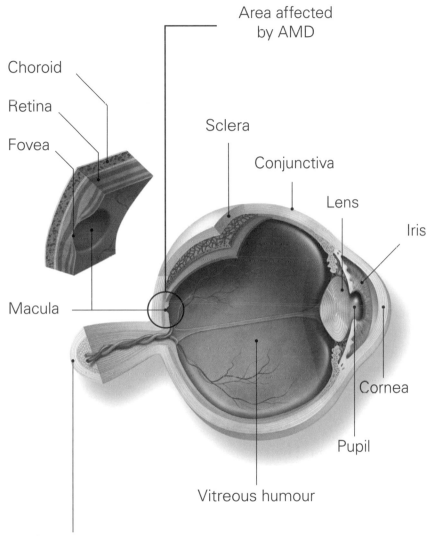

Area affected
by AMD

Choroid

Retina

Fovea

Sclera

Conjunctiva

Lens

Iris

Macula

Cornea

Optic nerve

Pupil

Vitreous humour

 Cross section of the eye

The sclera and the conjunctiva

The sclera (the white of the eye) is the tough outer wall that surrounds and protects the eye. The visible part of the sclera is covered by a thin, transparent membrane, the conjunctiva, which folds forward to become the lining of the inside of the eyelid.

The cornea

The cornea is the transparent membrane covering the eye, like the glass that covers the face of a watch. About a half millimetre thick, the cornea forms a clear dome over the iris, from which it is separated by aqueous fluid. The cornea controls the entry of light, protecting the inside of the eye against ultraviolet rays.

The iris and the pupil

At the centre of the iris (the part that gives the eye its colour) is an opening, the pupil, which allows light to enter the eye and reach the retina. The pupil contracts and dilates to control the amount of light that reaches the retina.

The lens

The lens is located behind the iris. The role of the lens is to focus images projected onto the back of the eye. To do this, the lens changes shape depending on the distance between the eye and the object viewed. With age, the lens loses its flexibility and cannot change shape as easily. This results it presbyopia, an inability to see near objects clearly without glasses. A cataract is an area of the lens that has become opaque.

The vitreous humour
Between the lens and the retina there is compartment containing a transparent jelly-like substance called the vitreous humour, or vitreous body, which enables the eyeball to hold its spherical shape.

The retina
The retina is a thin film of nerve tissue lining 75 percent of the inner surface of the eyeball. Here is where the photoreceptors are located, the cells that convert light to nerve impulses delivered to the brain by the optic nerve. AMD affects a very small part of the retina, the macula.

The macula
The macula is a very small area (about 2 mm in diameter) at the centre of the retina. The macula transmits 90 percent of the visual information processed by the brain. Composed of closely-packed visual cells, the macula is responsible for fine-detail vision (such as reading and recognizing faces) as well as colour detection. The retina as a whole allows us to see the book on the table, for example, but the macula makes it possible for us to read the words in the book. The macula is also called the "yellow spot" because of its yellow colour, due to a high concentration of lutein, an antioxidant of the carotenoid family.

The fovea
The fovea is a small dimple a half millimetre in diameter at the centre of the macula, the region of greatest visual acuity. The fovea is the centre of the eye's sharpest vision. It is also largely responsible for colour vision, thanks to its densely

packed cones (photoreceptors). The closer a lesion is to the fovea, the more devastating the central vision loss.

The optic nerve

Located at the back of the eye, the optic nerve transmits visual information to the brain. It is composed of roughly one million nerve fibres coming from the retina.

HOW WE SEE

Light passes first through the cornea, the aqueous humour, the lens and the vitreous humour before falling on the retina. It is there, not in the brain, that processing of the image by the nervous system begins. In fact, many anatomists consider the retina an extension of the brain.

As thin as a sheet of paper, the retina is nonetheless more complex and more sensitive than photographic film. It has ten distinct layers, each with a specific function. Light must cross several of these layers to reach the 125 million photoreceptors (light-sensitive cells) that absorb the light and convert it to nerve impulses, which are relayed to the brain via the optic nerve (*Figure* ❷).

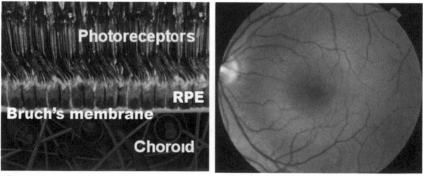

❷ Normal retina

The role of the photoreceptors

The retina contains two types of photoreceptors (rods and cones), and each plays a different role in the perception of images.

There are approximately 120 million rods in each eye, and they are sensitive to dim light, allowing us to see at night. During the day, or in bright light, the rods stop responding. Rods cannot resolve fine detail or distinguish colours, but they are responsible for peripheral vision.

There are fewer cones (five million), but their capacity to distinguish detail is one hundred times greater than that of the rods. Very numerous in the macula, cones are responsible for colour vision and are used mainly in bright light (during the day or with artificial lighting). Cones are tuned to different portions of the colour spectrum: some perceive blue, others red and still others green.

The photoreceptors use retinene (or retinal), a light-sensitive derivative of vitamin A, to convert light energy into nerve energy. Once used, retinene loses its light sensitivity. As the body cannot manufacture vitamin A, the retinene is recycled. This is where the retinal pigment epithelium (RPE) comes into play.

The role of the retinal pigment epithelium (RPE)

The retinal pigment epithelium (RPE) is a single layer of cells under the retina. One of the roles of the RPE is to remove waste from the retina that is produced by the photoreceptors when converting light to nerve impulses. AMD arises when the RPE starts to deteriorate. The deterioration spreads to the retina, particularly the macula, where the photosensitive cones responsible for central visual acuity and colour perception are located—causing central vision to become less clear and more and more blurry.

The role of the choroid
Located under the retina, between the RPE and the sclera, the choroid supplies the photoreceptors with the oxygen and nourishment they require to function properly. Though relatively small (a single layer of organic tissue), the choroid is composed mainly of blood vessels. The blood flow through these vessels is greater than anywhere else in the body, demonstrating the extent to which the photoreceptors need nourishment to function properly. Wet AMD is caused by the development of new abnormal vessels in the choroid (neovascularization). Fluid leaking from these abnormal vessels causes image distortion and loss of central vision.

The role of Bruch's membrane
Bruch's membrane is composed of five very thin layers. Located between the RPE and the choroid and physically separating the two structures, Bruch's membrane nonetheless allows metabolic exchanges between the photoreceptors, the RPE and the blood flow from the choroid (oxygen, nourishment and waste). In people with AMD, Bruch's membrane is abnormally thick from accumulation of drusen.

References
1. Pascolini D, Mariotti SP, Pokharel GP, et al. 2002 Global update of available data on visual impairment: a compilation of population-based prevalence studies, *Ophthalmic Epidemiol,* 2004;11:67-115.
2. CNIB
3. AMD Alliance International
4. Friedman DS, O'Colmain BJ, Muñoz B, et al. Prevalence of age-related macular degeneration in the United States. *Arch Ophthalmol,* 2004;122(4):564-72.

CHAPTER 2
THE TWO FORMS
OF AMD

Two different forms of AMD can affect the macula: wet AMD and dry AMD. The dry form is more common, accounting for 85 to 90 percent of AMD diagnoses. Dry AMD progresses slowly and rarely causes major vision loss. It generally affects both eyes, though not to the same degree or at the same rate.

The wet form of AMD derives its name from the fluid and blood that leak into the macula from abnormal blood vessels growing beneath it. The wet form of AMD accounts for only 10 to 15 percent of AMD cases, but it develops rapidly and can cause vision impairment within weeks if not days.

DRY AMD

Early signs

One of the earliest signs of the dry form of AMD is the appearance of small, round yellow deposits in Bruch's membrane. These are called drusen and they show up in an ocular fundus examination, that is, an examination of the back of the eye (*Figure❶*).

Composed mainly of proteins and fats, drusen are accumulations of waste products from cell activity. In absorbing light to convert it to nerve impulses, the photoreceptors produce waste. This waste is normally eliminated by the retinal pigment epithelium (RPE), which functions as the retina's refuse collector, among other things. Scientists still do not know why this debris accumulates. Perhaps the RPE is no longer able to do its job properly, or perhaps it is overworked because there is just too much waste. In any case, changes to the RPE are often observed in the early stages of the disease. Other hypotheses implicate Bruch's membrane, which, for reasons not understood, may become less permeable, inhibiting exchanges between the RPE and the choroid, particularly those required to eliminate waste (*see Chapter 3*).

If a vision specialist finds a few drusen in an eye, there is not necessarily cause for alarm. These deposits often form with age and their presence does not automatically indicate AMD. Drusen are like wrinkles—most people over 60 can expect to have some—but their progression must be monitored by an optometrist or an ophthalmologist.

Not all drusen are alike. Small drusen with well-defined borders are often harmless or signal a very early form of AMD—so early that it is sometimes impossible to tell if AMD is actually present. Large drusen with ill-defined bor-

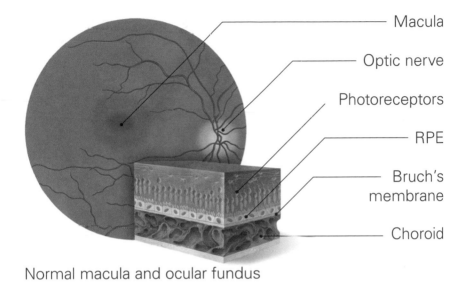

Macula
Optic nerve
Photoreceptors
RPE
Bruch's membrane
Choroid

Normal macula and ocular fundus

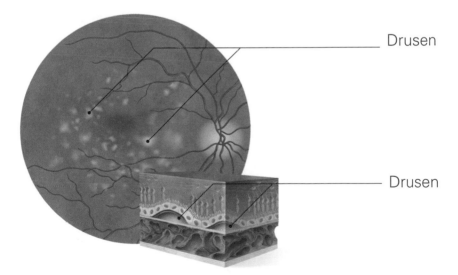

Drusen

Drusen

Macula and ocular fundus with drusen

1

ders, on the other hand, are an unequivocal indication of AMD. However, they must be located in the macula, which, as mentioned earlier, is responsible for colour and detailed vision. Drusen can also appear elsewhere in the retina (outside the macula), but in these locations they have virtually no impact on vision.

Drusen can remain unchanged for years ... or they can change. They may increase in number, develop ill-defined borders or spread to form large plaques in Bruch's membrane.

When this happens, Bruch's membrane can no longer do its job, causing disturbances in the transport of oxygen and nourishment between the retinal pigment epithelium (RPE), located just below the membrane, and the choroid, located just above it. Presence of drusen is also associated with changes to the cells of the RPE: photoreceptors that depend on proper functioning of the RPE for their survival will end up dying, causing a decline in vision quality.

How vision is affected

In the beginning, the changes are almost imperceptible. As dry AMD progresses slowly (over 10, 20 and sometimes even 30 years), substantial visual acuity may be lost in the affected eye without it being noticed; the eye that is not affected and the brain, which interprets the visual signals sent by the photoreceptors, together compensate for the vision loss.

There are, however, a few telling symptoms. More light may be needed to read and there may be difficulty adjusting to changes in light intensity. Contrast sensitivity and the ability to distinguish colours may decline (*Figure* ❷).

Reading can become more difficult, even with correctly prescribed glasses. People will say, "I can see, but I can't

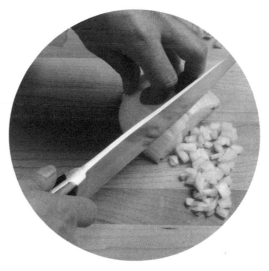

Normal vision

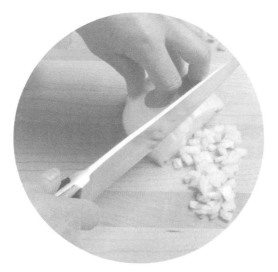

Diminished contrast sensitivity

❷

make out details." The more the drusen spread through the macula, the greater the risk of deterioration of central vision. Straight lines appear wavy and objects seem distorted. This is called metamorphopsia.

In the late stages of AMD (fortunately more rare), parts of the macula atrophy, preventing it from working properly. Small blurry or dark spots, called scotoma, then appear in the visual field, resulting in blind spots in the central vision. This is called atrophic AMD. When a large part of the macula has atrophied, we speak of advanced dry AMD. Advanced dry AMD can cause as much vision impairment as wet AMD, but its progression is much slower. However, even in the most advanced stages, all the changes that occur in the macula are completely painless (*Figure* ❸).

It is also encouraging that lifestyle changes, quitting smoking in particular, can very probably slow the progression of dry AMD, as we will see later.

WET AMD

Wet AMD only develops in people who already have dry AMD. This form of AMD is called wet or exudative AMD because of the growth of small abnormal blood vessels (neovascularization) that leak blood or fluid into the macula, causing hemorrhage or swelling.

According to the Age-Related Eye Disease Study (AREDS), a major study published by the National Eye Institute in the United States in 2002, only 1.3 percent of people with early stage dry AMD progress to the wet form or to advanced dry AMD.

The onset of the wet form of AMD can be very sudden, causing severe damage within days. Luckily this form of

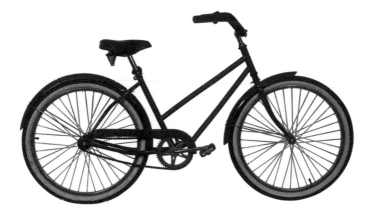

Normal vision

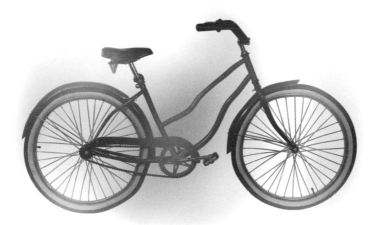

Vision with dry AMD

AMD is more rare, but it is responsible for 90 percent of severe central vision loss due to AMD.

Signs of progression to wet AMD

We still do not understand what causes dry AMD to turn into wet AMD. However, it has been established that growth of abnormal blood vessels (neovascularization) under the retina is associated with secretion of a substance called vascular endothelial growth factor, or VEGF, by certain retinal cells. These abnormal blood vessels have fragile walls that leak fluid or blood, causing swelling and tiny hemorrhages in the retina (*Figure* ❹).

SYMPTOMS OF WET AMD AND DRY AMD

A number of symptoms may appear, together or alone, when AMD progresses. These are the most common:

• Need for more light when reading

• Loss of contrast sensitivity

• Distortion of straight lines (metamorphopsia)

• Loss of visual acuity, manifested as difficulty recognizing faces or distinguishing letters on a page

• Diminished colour perception

• Appearance of blurry or dark spots (scotoma) in the central visual field

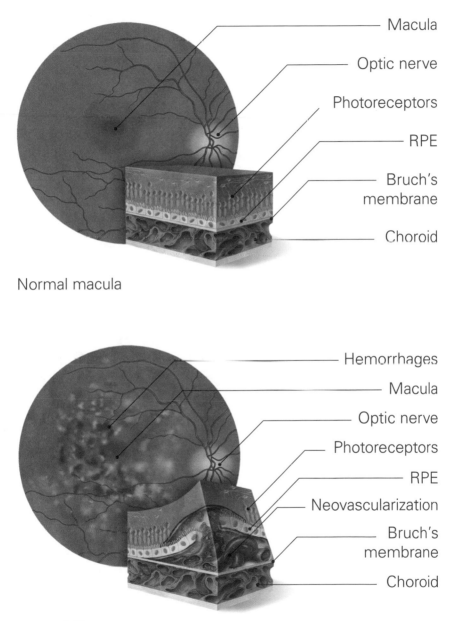

Macula

Optic nerve

Photoreceptors

RPE

Bruch's membrane

Choroid

Normal macula

Hemorrhages

Macula

Optic nerve

Photoreceptors

RPE

Neovascularization

Bruch's membrane

Choroid

Wet AMD

How vision is affected

In an area as small and complex as the macula, even a very small leak will damage the photoreceptors and prevent the transmission of visual signals. Straight lines may start to appear wavy or irregular (metamorphopsia), and blurry spots may appear in the central visual field (*Figure* ❺).

The presence of blood and fluid unfortunately provokes a tissue repair process that modifies the anatomy and function of the retina. In other words, in the absence or failure of treatment, a scar will form in the macula, causing vision impairment.

Even though blurry spots can also appear in dry AMD, they develop much more quickly in wet AMD. Without treatment, central vision can disappear entirely, at a pace that varies from one individual to the next—making it very difficult, if not impossible, to read or drive a car. In addition, when exudative (wet) AMD develops in one eye, the risk of its developing in the other eye is high. Thankfully, there are measures that can be taken to seal the leaky blood vessels and inhibit their proliferation before the damage gets worse (*see Chapter 5*).

THE STAGES OF AMD

AMD is currently divided into four stages, though the symptoms listed may vary from one person to the next.

Early AMD

Several small drusen appear in the retina of one eye (more often both eyes). However, central vision is the same as in people who do not have AMD.

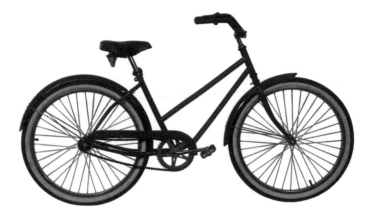

Normal vision

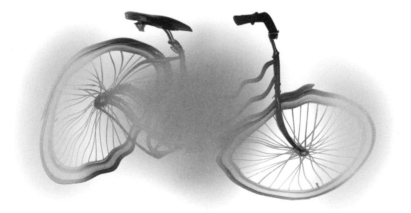

Vision with wet AMD

5

Intermediate AMD

There are many medium-sized drusen or one or more large drusen in one or both eyes. Straight lines may appear wavy but there is no major vision loss.

Advanced dry AMD

The photoreceptors of the macula stop working properly. A blurry or dark spot appears in the centre of vision. At this stage, the risk of developing wet AMD is high.

Wet AMD

Parts of the macula are invaded by fluid and blood. The photoreceptors are damaged, causing blurry or dark spots to appear in central vision. Once wet AMD has developed in one eye, there is a 50 percent chance of its developing in the other eye within five years.

DON'T DESPAIR ...

A diagnosis of AMD comes as a shock. The most common questions are "Will I go blind?" and "Will I still be able to read or drive my car." But don't panic. AMD has several stages and it develops differently depending on the person.

Most people diagnosed with AMD have the dry form, which is less aggressive. In fact, in some people dry AMD progresses very little for years. In addition, lifestyle changes (and in some cases, appropriate nutritional supplements) can slow the progression of the disease and minimize the risk of conversion to wet AMD.

And even those with advanced AMD diagnosed at a late stage never go completely blind. In a worst-case scenario, central vision may disappear, but sight is never completely lost. Peripheral vision, ensured by the rest of the retina, is not affected by AMD. This means it is still possible to get about alone and remain independent. In addition, with the help of vision aids, it is very often possible to continue one's activities and enjoy life.

ONE PERSON'S STORY

Name: Simone	**Age:** 78

Occupation: Retired journalist

At 78 years of age, Simone had been followed for dry AMD for 11 years. She lived alone in her apartment, and her disease did not interfere with her daily activities. "I babysat my grandchildren occasionally, I did my own grocery shopping, cooking and housework, even though my central vision had diminished slightly over the years," she explains. One morning, Simone realized that vision in her right eye had deteriorated considerably. There was a dark spot and images were distorted. This had never happened before. "I was very worried, even though I had been assured that AMD would never cause me to go blind."

The optometrist who examined Simone confirmed that vision in her right eye had declined substantially since her last examination. He checked to make sure this wasn't due to a cataract or an inappropriate eyeglass correction, and he examined the back of her eye (the ocular fundus). He discovered that Simone had developed the wet form of AMD in her right eye, where blood was visible in the fundus. Simone quickly obtained an appointment with her ophthalmologist, who confirmed these findings and ordered fluorescein angiography. This examination was followed by monthly intraocular injections of ranibizumab (Lucentis®). After six months, the blood had completely disappeared and

Simone had recovered most of the vision she had lost as a result of the hemorrhage. She is being followed closely and will receive other injections if necessary. Simone is thrilled: "I'm very happy that I've been able to remain independent," she says with delight.

CHAPTER 3
RISK FACTORS

When diagnosed with a disease, we inevitably search for a culprit—the deciding factor, the mistake we made. Research has not yet made it possible to identify the causes of AMD with any certainty. There are a number of risk factors that may be responsible for onset of the disease—age and family history being the main ones, and the best known. It is thought, however, that certain behaviours or habits may increase the risk of developing AMD.

A WORD ABOUT CAUSES

We do not know why accumulations of debris appear in Bruch's membrane. Some scientists think that an overabundance of free radicals may be the cause. All cells in the human body generate energy from the oxygen we inhale and the food we eat, and this produces waste in the form of free radicals. A large quantity of free radicals are produced in the macula in particular, because the photoreceptors need a lot of oxygen to do their work of converting light into nerve signals that the brain can interpret. The body has an excellent defence system to keep free radicals in check: it uses antioxidants (such as vitamin C, vitamin E, beta carotene and zinc) derived from the food we eat.

Unfortunately, as we age, our bodies produce more free radicals than we are able to neutralize—especially with excessive sun exposure, smoking and consumption of trans or saturated fats. The problem is aggravated if our diets do not contain sufficient antioxidants. This may explain the accumulation of debris on Bruch's membrane: with too many free radicals, the retinal pigment epithelium (RPE) is not up to the task and is no longer able to clear away the waste.

Inflammation may also play a role. An inflammatory reaction is the body's response to aggression, part of its defence system. For example, infection by bacteria sets an army of proteins in motion to fight the infection. Once the infection is under control, other proteins set to work to calm the inflammation. In some families, however, the proteins that play this antiinflammatory role don't work properly because of a genetic variation—leading to exaggerated inflammatory responses such as allergies or rheumatoid arthritis.

Genetic abnormalities of the immune system (particularly of the complement system, a group of proteins that provoke an inflammatory reaction) may prove to be predisposing factors in AMD as well. Dysfunction of Complement Factor H (CFH), a complement system protein whose job is to control inflammation, plays a key role in the development (pathogenesis) of AMD and has as a result become an important target for future new therapies.

WHAT DOES NOT CAUSE AMD

We've all heard if from our grandmothers: "You'll ruin your eyes with all that reading!" However, there is no scientific basis to this common belief. Our eyes don't wear out any more quickly from reading than from looking out the window. AMD is not caused by reading too much or by spending too much time in front of the computer or sewing. And continuing these activities after a diagnosis of AMD does not make the disease worse.

It is clear that certain lifestyle habits can damage the eyes—such as spending long days under bright sunlight without sunglasses. This bad habit can increase the risk of cataracts and perhaps even AMD.

RISK FACTORS

Though we are still waiting to pinpoint the exact causes of AMD, we have identified factors that increase the risks of its development. Scientists generally believe that AMD is triggered when the combined effect of diverse risk factors crosses a threshold. At present, there are certain known risk factors for AMD and other probable risk factors.

We have no control over some of these risk factors, such as age and family history. However, others can be controlled: smoking, a diet poor in fruits and vegetables and a sedentary lifestyle. Nonetheless, as with all health problems, there are people with these risk factors who never develop AMD, whereas others who do not seem predisposed to it do.

Known risk factors

Age

Though the figures vary, all studies indicate that the risk of developing AMD increases with age. AMD rarely occurs before age 50 and mainly affects people over 65. After age 75, the risk of developing AMD increases dramatically.

Family history

Family history is another major risk factor. Studies indicate that the risk of developing AMD increases fourfold if a close family member (father, mother, brother or sister) has it.

PREVALENCE BY AGE AMONG CAUCASIANS*

Early AMD
Age 49-54: 1.3% to 9.4%
Age 55-64: 2.4% to 16.3%
Age 65-74: 8.5% to 24%
Age 75-84: 13.5% to 36.3%
Age 85 and over: 18.2% to 40.6%

Advanced AMD
Age 49-54: 0% to 0.1%
Age 55-64: 0.1% to 0.5%
Age 65-74: 0.7% to 1.4%
Age 75-84: 3.2% to 6.9%
Age 85 and over: 11.6% to 18.5%

* According to the Beaver Dam (U.S., 1993), Rotterdam (Netherlands, 2001) and Blue Mountains (Australia, 2002) studies.

Smoking

On this question, all researchers agree: smoking is by far the most important modifiable factor. Smokers are three times more likely to develop dry AMD than nonsmokers and six times more at risk for developing wet AMD. One possible explanation is that smoking generates a lot of free radicals. In addition, nicotine, a component of tobacco, is an angiogenic agent, which means it stimulates the development of neovascularization—a key factor in the wet form of AMD.

Sex

Though we don't know why, the risk of developing AMD is slightly higher in women than in men.

Race

Light-skinned people are more likely to develop AMD than those who are dark-skinned. Caucasians are twice as likely to develop AMD as black people.

Probable risk factors

A diet poor in fruits and vegetables

A diet low in fruits and vegetables is another risk factor. The correlation between smoking, exposure to bright light, age and AMD suggests the disease results from an excess of free radicals. Fruits and vegetables are rich in antioxidants, which are known to neutralize free radicals.

Excessive exposure to bright light

Repeated exposure to bright light may also play a role in the onset of AMD—blue light in particular, which is part of the spectrum of sunlight and is reflected on snow or water. Bright light makes the photoreceptors work harder and causes them to produce more waste. The retinal pigment epithelium, which is responsible for removing such waste, may not be able to keep up.

Obesity

Studies show that people who are obese are at higher risk of developing AMD. In addition, a diet rich in saturated fats and trans fats also increases the risk of developing AMD.

Blue or light iris colour

According to some studies, blue or light iris colour (blues, greens, greys) increases the risk, as these irises contain less pigment and allow more light to enter the eye than darker irises. However, prolonged and repeated exposure to bright light can contribute to the onset of AMD

Presence of other diseases

Untreated high blood pressure, atherosclerosis, high cholesterol and a family history of heart disease are other risk factors.

Cataract surgery

According to some scientists, cataract surgery can aggravate existing AMD. Other scientists, however, do not agree. Further studies are required to clarify this issue.

ONE PERSON'S STORY

Name: John	**Age:** 58

Occupation: Sales representative

At age 58, John was a sales representative for a major manufacturer of doors and windows. Shopping at the supermarket in his neighbourhood one day after work, he noticed that he was having difficulty reading prices on food items. Blaming fatigue, John didn't react right away. When he finally realized that his vision wasn't returning to normal and that he was needing more light to read, he made an appointment with the optometrist.

"I wasn't really surprised to find out I had AMD, because my father and brother had already been diagnosed with it," says John. John was referred to an ophthalmologist, who performed a fundus examination and fluorescein angiography before telling him that he had dry AMD and was at risk for developing the wet form of the disease. "My family history and the presence of drusen on my macula confirmed the diagnosis," he explains. His doctor convinced him to put all the odds in his favour and quit smoking, change his diet and take daily vitamin supplements (no beta carotenes).

"I wanted to preserve my sight as long as possible and continue working, so I followed all of my ophthalmologists recommendations. The hardest thing was to quit

smoking, but I had been considering it for a long time."
With these lifestyle changes, John has reduced the risk
of his dry AMD converting to the wet form. "And I feel
so much healthier!" he adds.

CHAPTER 4
DIAGNOSIS

Many health practitioners play a role in evaluating and monitoring eye and vision problems. Both optometrists and ophthalmologists are qualified to detect AMD. An examination of the back of the eye (fundus examination) is required for a diagnosis to be made. After that, the ophthalmologist uses a variety of tests, performed in a private clinic or hospital, to determine the form of AMD (wet or dry) and appropriate therapy.

EARLY DETECTION

Early detection of AMD is crucial, so treatment can begin as soon as possible when indicated.

Seeing straight lines as wavy (metamorphopsia) is often an early sign of the wet form of AMD, especially when it happens suddenly. People with wet AMD also tend to see one or more blurry or dark spots, because of the presence of blood or fluid under the macula. These symptoms may also occur in advanced dry AMD, when parts of the macula atrophy.

Anyone experiencing these symptoms is strongly advised to consult a doctor as soon as possible.

We cannot emphasize enough the importance of regular eye examinations, even if there does not seem to be any deterioration of vision. AMD-related changes can be detected in a routine eye examination even before symptoms appear.

COMPREHENSIVE EYE EXAMINATION

As part of the eye examination, a technician or vision specialist (optometrist or ophthalmologist) takes note of past health problems and performs certain tests. There are several steps before the back of the eye is examined (fundus examination).

General health and eye health questionnaire

In addition to recent symptoms, it is important to know the patient's state of health (diabetes, high blood pressure, heart disease, allergies, etc.), family history and any treatment or medication he or she is taking.

Visual acuity test

Vision is measured using a visual acuity chart called the Snellen chart or scale. The chart consists of rows of letters or drawings that decrease in size line by line. Vision specialists are referring to this chart when they speak of a gain or loss of a "line of visual acuity."

Visual acuity tests measure the sharpness of central vision, needed for seeing details clearly. Visual acuity scores are expressed as a fraction not a percentage.

Normal vision is 6/6 (in metres) or (20/20) (in feet). The first number of the fraction represents the distance of the patient from the Snellen chart. The second number shows the distance from which most people without a visual impairment would be able to read the line of letters on the chart.

VISUAL IMPAIRMENT

Anyone whose visual acuity with an adequate optical correction is less than 6/21 (or 20/70) has a major visual impairment. This means the person can see at six metres (or 20 feet) an object that is generally perceived at 21 metres (or 70 feet) by someone with perfect vision.

If central vision is 6/60 (20/200) or less, the person is considered "legally blind."

Eye examination

An eye examination will show if there are other causes of diminished vision, such as cataracts, glaucoma or other eye diseases. It includes an external examination of the eye and its adnexa (eyelids, tear glands and tear ducts), an evaluation of ocular motility (an eye that deviates, excessive movement, etc.), a biomicroscopic examination (for detecting cataracts, vitreous hemorrhage, etc.) and intraocular pressure measurement.

WHO DOES WHAT

• An optician makes and sells corrective lenses based on a prescription written by an optometrist or an ophthalmologist. Opticians do not perform eye examinations.

• Optometrists are vision professionals but are not physicians. They are often the first practitioner consulted when vision problems arise. Based on a clinical eye examination, an optometrist can identify certain eye and vision problems, prescribe and/or sell glasses and, if need be, refer the patient to an ophthalmologist.

• An ophthalmologist is a medical doctor. He or she is trained to perform a complete assessment of visual function, make diagnoses and provide medical and surgical treatment of diseases or disorders of the eye and related structures (eyelids, tear glands and tear ducts).

Fundus examination

A diagnosis of AMD is made by an optometrist or an ophthalmologist based on an examination of the back of the eye (the fundus), which makes it possible to evaluate the condition of the retina. There are different ways of performing this examination: it can be done with an ophthalmoscope or a biomicroscope (slit-lamp), with or without contact lenses. The patient's pupil must be dilated.

A fundus examination is not painful. It allows the vision specialist to see characteristic signs of AMD, such as presence of drusen, irregularities in the deep layer of the retina or more serious lesions (changes to the pigment epithelium, hemorrhage or lipid deposits). The vision specialist will also be able to see the characteristics of the drusen—if they have ill-defined or well-defined borders and if they are numerous. With this information, the type of AMD (wet or dry) can generally be determined, and a decision can be made about what to do next (*Figure* ❶).

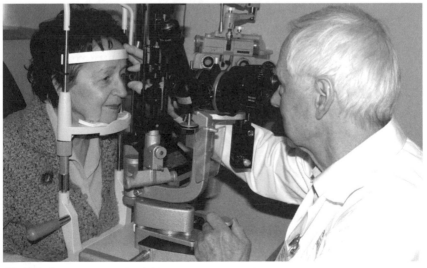

❶ Slit-lamp examination

FUNDUS AUTOFLUORESENCE

This examination is not often performed, but it can tell the ophthalmologist about the progression of dry AMD.

Fundus autofluorescence takes advantage of the fluorescent properties of certain substances—lipofuscin in particular, a cellular pigment composed of molecular debris. Lipofuscin is naturally present in the ocular fundus, particularly in the retinal pigment epithelium (RPE). Autofluorescence is strong in dry AMD and disappears completely where there is RPE loss in atrophic zones (atrophic AMD).

To perform the examination, light is sent to the back of the eye. The tissue then emits autofluorescence and photographic images of the fundus autofluorescence are obtained using a variety of angiographic devices equipped with special filters. The pupil must be dilated for this examination.

FLUORESCEIN ANGIOGRAPHY

Fluorescein angiography is a technique for examining blood circulation of the retina by injecting a dye (fluorescein or indocyanine green) into a vein. This test can be used to find out if a patient has dry or wet AMD (*Figure ❷*). It also confirms the presence and scope of neovascularization (growth of abnormal blood vessels) and the location of the new blood vessels. Well-defined neovascularization on the RPE is called classic neovascularization. Neovascularization that is under the RPE and not well-delineated is called occult neovascularization.

For this test, like the fundus examination, the pupil is dilated with eye drops. The dye injected into a vein in the patient's forearm or hand quickly reaches the eye and colours

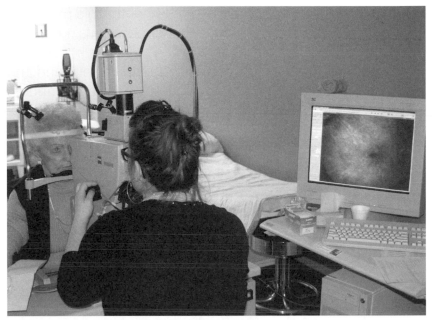

Fluorescein angiography equipment

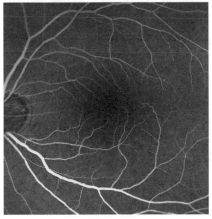

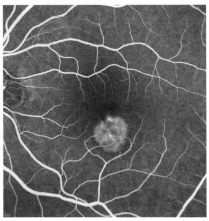

Normal angiogram

Abnormal angiogram
(neovascularization)

the vessels at the back of the eye. The ophthalmic photographer or technician then takes a series of photos using a camera equipped with special filters.

Fluorescein is the dye most frequently used, and the examination takes only a few minutes. It is rarely necessary to use indocyanine green, which allows examination of deeper layers (choroid).

Adverse effects of dyes

Adverse effects of angiography are rare and generally not harmful. Fluorescein can provoke nausea, dizziness and sometimes vomiting. When these effects occur, they do so in within minutes of the injection of the dye and disappear just as rapidly.

Strong allergic reactions to fluorescein (anaphylaxis) are extremely rare.

Fluorescein in the blood stream colours the skin and the whites of the eyes an orangey yellow. This discoloration appears a few minutes after the dye is injected and lasts for several hours. The urine will also appear dark yellow or orange for about 24 hours.

Indocyanine green is well tolerated and does not cause nausea or vomiting. However, as it contains iodine, it must not be given to anyone with an iodine allergy. In addition, it is not recommended in the first three months of pregnancy.

Indocyanine green causes stools to turn green.

PUPIL DILATION

Pupil dilation is required for a proper fundus examination as well as for fluorescein angiography and fundus autofluorescence. Drops are put in the eye to force the pupil to stay open. It takes about 15 minutes for the drops to take full effect. Pupil dilation is not painful, but the eyes may become sensitive to light and near vision can be disturbed for several hours. It is thus recommended that the patient bring a pair of sunglasses and either be accompanied or make arrangements for the trip home. Patients are advised not to drive for several hours after the examination.

OPTICAL COHERENCE TOMOGRAPHY (OCT)

Optical coherence tomography, or OCT, is like an ultrasound, except light is used instead of sound. The OCT scanner measures the speed of light traveling through the ocular media and the retina and the time it takes for the light to be reflected back by tissues and structures. These measurements are used to generate cross-sectional images of the back of the eye (the ocular fundus), from the outermost to the deepest layers.

OCT is used to measure the thickness of the retina. Within minutes, macular edema caused by accumulation of fluid or blood can be detected, painlessly and without injection, and its location within or under the retina pinpointed.

OCT is currently used to diagnose and follow patients with AMD. It is very helpful in evaluating treatment efficacy. OCT provides information different from but complementary to that obtained from angiography (*Figure* ❸).

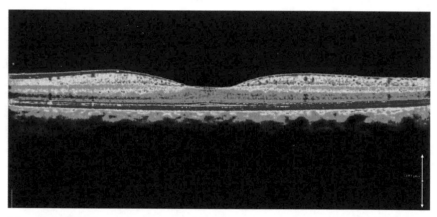

Normal OCT scan

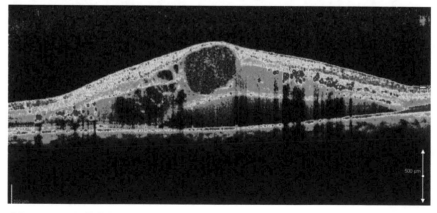

Abnormal OCT scan

❸

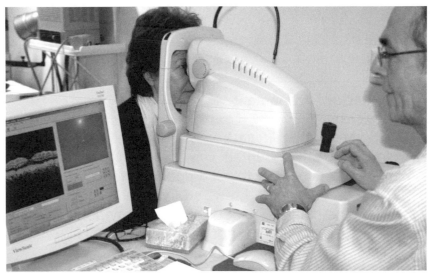

Optical coherence tomography (OCT) scanner

❸

ULTRASOUND

Eye ultrasounds are rarely necessary in AMD. They are only useful when media opacity (hemorrhage or cataract) makes it impossible to properly evaluate the ocular fundus with the other examinations.

ONE PERSON'S STORY

Name: Mark	**Age:** 56

Occupation: Accountant

At 56 years of age, Mark kept in shape with regular exercise. As an accountant, he spent long hours using his eyes continuously to read documents and work at the computer. "When I realized I was having difficulty reading fine print, I decided to consult my optometrist to get my eyeglass prescription checked," he explains.

The optometrist tested Mark's eyes and found his correction was perfect for far vision but an adjustment was required for close vision. During the visit, the optometrist also examined the back of Mark's eyes (ocular fundus examination). As a precaution, he referred Mark to an ophthalmologist. "My wife came with me, because the secretary warned me that my pupils would be dilated and I might not be able to drive home," says Mark. "I didn't know what to expect. I was afraid the examination would be painful and I was anxious. The ophthalmologist performed a fundus examination and fluorescein angiography. It was completely painless and only took a few minutes."

The diagnosis was early dry AMD. "I was completely devastated by the news," Mark recalls, "as I thought I was going to go blind. However, the ophthalmologist reassured me, explaining that my problem was minor and that all I needed was to take vitamin supplements."

Mark did not have to make any other lifestyle changes. He has his eyes checked regularly, and he knows that if his vision declines suddenly, he must consult his ophthalmologist rapidly for any necessary medical treatment.

CHAPTER 5

PREVENTION AND TREATMENT

Giant strides have been made in AMD research in the last ten years. Though scientists do not yet have all the answers, we have a better understanding of the disease. Nonetheless, there is still no cure. On the other hand, as AMD is being diagnosed earlier and earlier, we are sometimes able to slow the progression of the dry form. And for the wet form, we now have much more effective treatments to stabilize and sometimes even improve vision.

PREVENTING OR SLOWING THE PROGRESSION OF AMD

When a family member has AMD, we want to know what to do to avoid getting it too. And if we have received a diagnosis of AMD, we want to do everything possible to preserve our sight. Obviously, there is not much we can do about our genetics. However, we can act on the "modifiable" risk factors that promote onset or progression of AMD. Studies show that certain lifestyle changes can reduce the risks.

Quit smoking
Far less AMD is found in nonsmokers than in smokers. Not smoking definitely reduces the risk of onset or progression of AMD.

There are a number of effective methods of quitting. Your pharmacist or family doctor can tell you more.

Eat right
It's a fact: the rate of AMD is lower in people with diets rich in antioxidants—particularly dark green vegetables such as spinach. Conversely, levels of macular lutein, a yellow pigment present in the macula, are 32 percent lower in people with AMD than in people without it. In addition, a recent large-scale study showed that a diet rich in lutein significantly lowers the risk of developing wet AMD. Last, people who get sufficient dietary zinc (a trace element found in sizable quantities in meat, seafood, fish and nuts) are less likely to develop AMD than those who don't.

WHERE TO FIND ANTIOXIDANTS

Lutein and zeaxanthin
Lutein and zeaxanthin are antioxidants of the carotenoid family. They are found in kale, spinach, basil, parsley, peas, zucchini, leeks, lettuce, broccoli, corn, Brussels sprouts and asparagus.

Antioxidant vitamins
- Vitamin C: in citrus fruits (oranges, lemons, grapefruit), kiwi, broccoli, strawberries and peppers (yellow, green and red).
- Vitamin E: in wheat germ, nuts, peanut butter, sunflower seeds, papaya and avocado.
- Beta carotene: in chives, parsley, green onions, sweet potatoes, kale, pumpkin, spinach, peas and carrots.

Antioxidant minerals
- Zinc: in oysters, dark chocolate, beef, veal and lamb.
- Copper: in oysters, dark chocolate, lobster, nuts and liver (calf, beef and lamb).
- Selenium: in cod, mussels, tuna, mackerel, wheat flour, anchovies, grilled bacon, swordfish, sardines and kidney (pork, lamb and beef).

Take omega-3

There are no studies that clearly demonstrate the benefits of taking omega-3 in people with AMD. However, omega-3 fatty acids, particularly DHA (docosahexaenoic acid), are key components of retinal cells. In addition, AMD prevalence is lower in people who take omega-3.

Avoid saturated and trans fats

Vascular problems are often associated with consumption of saturated and trans fats. These two types of fat may thus have an impact on the progression of AMD.

Saturated fats are found mainly in meat and animal products: butter, cream, lard, animal fat. They are also found in certain plant-derived products, such as coconut oil and palm oil.

Trans fats are obtained from unsaturated vegetable oils (generally soybean, corn or canola oil). They make it possible to produce fats that can withstand high cooking temperatures and margarines with a long shelf-life that are solid at room temperature.

Trans fats increase the risk of developing AMD. They are found mainly in commercial fried foods and baked goods containing partially hydrogenated oils: cookies, crackers, doughnuts, cakes, pastries, muffins, croissants, snacks and fried or breaded foods. Watch out for waffles, pancakes, oriental noodles, snack puddings, popcorn, chips and cereal bars! Read labels carefully and look for labels that say "no trans fats."

Protect your eyes from bright light

Bright light, natural as well as artificial, makes the retinal pigment epithelium and the photoreceptors work harder. It is important to wear sunglasses to prevent extended exposure to glare as much as possible—especially light reflecting off snow, sand or water.

Watch your weight

The risk of developing AMD is higher in people who are overweight. Regular exercise is important and the recommendations in *Canada's Food Guide* should be followed. This will protect your heart as well.

Have your eyes examined regularly

The Canadian Ophthalmological Society recommends the following frequencies for eye examinations by an ophthalmologist or an optometrist:

- Between age 41 and 50, every five years
- Between age 55 and 65, every three years
- After age 65, every two years

The ophthalmologist or optometrist decides the consultation frequency for people with AMD.

Keep cardiovascular disease under control

Cardiovascular problems can play a role in worsening AMD. Disorders such as high blood pressure, atherosclerosis, elevated cholesterol or heart disease should be monitored by your family doctor.

Use the Amsler grid

The Amsler grid is a square composed of thin lines in a grid formation that is used to monitor the onset of metamorphopsia, a visual distortion that causes straight lines to appear wavy. Metamorphopsia can indicate progression of AMD to a more advanced stage.

The Amsler grid is a very sensitive test. If you look at the grid for too long, no matter what the condition of your macula, your vision will end up blurry. The test should only take a few seconds. Each eye is checked separately, the other eye covered with your hand. If the straight lines seem bent or fuzzy, an eye specialist should be consulted without delay. The physician or optometrist decides how often the Amsler grid test should be performed, depending on the stage of AMD (*Figure* ❶).

Take food supplements

The Age-Related Eye Disease Study (AREDS) published by the U.S. National Eye Institute in 2001 demonstrated that people with intermediate or advanced AMD were less likely to develop a more advanced form of the disease if they took vitamin E and C, beta carotene and zinc supplements. The risk of dry AMD worsening or converting to wet AMD was 25 percent lower among study participants taking supplements than among those not taking them. Central vision loss attributable to AMD also dropped by 19 percent. People with AMD are thus strongly advised to take nutritional supplements regularly, unless counselled otherwise by their doctor.

One cautionary note: an increased incidence of lung cancer has been noted in smokers who take beta carotene supplements.

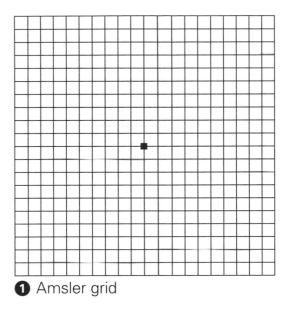

❶ Amsler grid

A doctor or an optometrist is the best person to recommend vitamin supplements formulated according to the conclusions of the AREDS study. These tablets are specially designed for people with intermediate or advanced AMD, as dosages are much higher than in standard multivitamins. The AREDS study did not demonstrate that such dosages are beneficial for people who don't have AMD or have early AMD. It is always best to check with your pharmacist about possible interactions with other medication you may be taking.

Two other antioxidants will be covered in the conclusions of the AREDS 2 study, the results of which will be known in 2012. These are lutein and zeaxanthin, carotenoid pigments naturally present in the macula that filter out most blue light before it reaches the photoreceptors. While awaiting the results of this prospective study, a number of manufacturers are already including lutein and zeaxanthin in their nutritional supplement formulations. Also, pharmaceutical companies are now adding omega-3 to their formulations in addition to these antioxidants.

TREATING DRY AMD

Scientists have not yet succeeded in developing effective treatments for dry AMD. Attempts have been made (such as using a laser to eliminate drusen), but without success. However, intensive research is being conducted, and major discoveries are expected in the near future (*see Chapter 7*). At the moment, prevention through healthy lifestyle choices is the best way to preserve vision quality if you have dry AMD. If you have intermediate or advanced AMD, nutritional supplements formulated based on the AREDS results must be taken to limit progression of the disease.

TREATING WET AMD

Laser therapy

Considerable progress has been made over the last 10 years in the treatment of wet AMD. Until the turn of the century, the main treatment was laser photocoagulation to seal the neovascularization. The laser emits light that turns to heat when absorbed by the retina. The heat closes off the unwanted blood vessels, stopping the leakage of blood and fluid. Unfortunately, the laser beam also burns a scar in the macula, causing vision loss in the treated area. In addition, the laser burns not only abnormal blood vessels but also surrounding healthy tissue.

DON'T BE TAKEN IN!

Ozone therapy, magnetic therapy, herbal treatments, energy rebalancing therapy, fat tissue transplants to the eye ... despite all the promises, there is currently no scientific evidence that these therapies have any value in the treatment of AMD. The same is true for acupuncture, rheopheresis and homeopathic remedies. They do not improve vision or cure AMD. A treatment must be scientifically proven and clinically tested before it is prescribed to patients. When someone suggests an extraordinary therapy that no doctor has ever heard of, one should be suspicious. If some miraculous cure has been discovered, the doctor will be among the first to know!

Though laser photocoagulation destroys existing neovascularization, in 50 percent of cases new abnormal blood vessels appear. For these reasons, laser photocoagulation is no longer used to treat wet AMD. It is, however, used with success to treat other eye diseases, such as diabetic retinopathy.

Photodynamic therapy (PDT)

Developed in the early part of the century, this treatment uses a non-thermal laser beam together with a light-activated drug. Here is how the treatment is administered: The patient receives a 10-minute intravenous injection of verteporfin (Visudyne®), a light-activated drug. The drug travels through the bloodstream and collects in the abnormal blood vessels in the retina. The doctor then puts anesthetic drops in the patient's eye to minimize discomfort and places a special lens over the eye so the area to be treated can be clearly seen.

Five minutes after the intravenous injection, the doctor activates a cold (non-thermal) laser beam, illuminating the verteporfin in the abnormal blood vessels for 83 seconds. The treatment seals the abnormal blood vessels by provoking photothrombosis. In other words, blood clots form in the abnormal vessels, closing them off without destroying vision. The procedure is generally painless.

The patient is more sensitive to sunlight and bright light for 48 hours after the treatment. To prevent photosensitivity, the patient must wear a hat, sunglasses and clothing that covers the skin entirely if he or she goes outside. It is best to remain indoors as much as possible and to avoid sources of bright light, such as halogen lamps.

The efficacy of photodynamic therapy is recognized. The problem is that, as with laser photocoagulation, the destruction of existing neovascularization does not prevent recurrence. Vascular endothelial growth factor (VEGF) continues to stimulate the proliferation of new abnormal blood vessels, which means the treatment must be repeated every three months.

Today, photodynamic therapy alone is rarely used to treat wet AMD. New drugs, antiangiogenic agents, are used as well. Studies currently in progress are measuring the efficacy of combining photodynamic therapy and antiangiogenic drugs.

Antiangiogenic drugs

A major breakthrough was made in late 2004 in the treatment of wet AMD. Thanks to the development of antiangiogenic agents, drugs that block neovascularization, we are finally able to neutralize vascular endothelial growth factor

(VEGF). To stop abnormal blood vessel growth, antiangiogenic drugs are injected directly into the eye. There are currently three antiangiogenic drugs available to treat wet AMD: ranibizumab (Lucentis®), pegaptanib (Macugen®) and bevacizumab (Avastin®). Of the three, only ranibizumab (Lucentis®) and pegaptanib (Macugen®) have been the subject of clinical studies with control groups (studies in which one group takes the drug and another does not) to evaluate their efficacy and safety. These studies clearly demonstrated the superiority of ranibizumab (Lucentis®) in preserving and even improving visual acuity in patients treated for wet AMD.

The treatment generally consists of a series of three or four monthly injections followed by another series of injections at intervals that depend on the patient's progress. To date, the best results have been obtained with monthly injections over two years. Ways to reduce the number of injections are being studied.

Treatment procedure

First, to reduce the risk of infection, patients are asked not to wear any make-up on the day of the treatment. An imaging test (OCT) is sometimes performed before the injection, so the doctor can assess the condition of the retina. The eye is then disinfected and anesthetized using drops or an injection. An eyelid speculum is used to hold the eyelid open, and the injection is administered into the white of the eye. The procedure is not painful and is well-tolerated. Slight bleeding under the conjunctiva of the eye and eye irritation are normal after the injection. To prevent infection, the patient must use antibiotic drops for a few days. The patient can return to work on the following day.

Encouraging results

Clinical studies conducted with ranibizumab (Lucentis®) demonstrated that after two years of monthly treatments vision stabilized in nine out of 10 patients, and one out of three patients gained three or more lines of visual acuity on the Snellen scale (see Chapter 4). By the end of the study, 40 percent of the patients with wet AMD had maintained sufficient visual acuity to keep their driver's license. One thing is certain: initial visual acuity, the size of the lesion and whether or not it affects the fovea (the centre of the macula) all have a bearing on the outcome of the treatment.

Combination therapies

Combination therapies that use photodynamic therapy, antiangiogenics and occasionally steroids (a form of cortisone) are sometimes employed to treat people with wet AMD. Such therapies are attractive because they reduce the number of procedures and doctor's visits while stabilizing vision. Studies are currently being conducted to find out if patients achieve the same visual acuity results with these combination therapies as with ranibizumab (Lucentis®) therapy alone—but with far fewer injections. It is important to remember that treatment frequency and type are personalized depending on the patient's age, general health and ability to travel as well as the condition of the other eye and other factors.

Radiation therapy

Studies of treatments that combine radiation therapy and injections of antiangiogenics are in progress. However, there are as yet no results to warrant clinical application of this type of treatment.

Surgery

There are no operations that can cure wet AMD. Surgery is rarely used to treat AMD, except in cases of major hemorrhage.

ONE PERSON'S STORY

Name: Paul	**Age:** 66

Occupation: Volunteer chauffeur

At age 66, Paul was a volunteer chauffeur for the handicapped. The vision in his right eye was very reduced due to advanced dry AMD and the vision in his left eye was 6/9 (20/30) due to early dry AMD. "One morning, I poured water but missed the glass and realized that the vision in my better eye had suddenly declined. I also noticed that the objects around me seemed distorted," he explains. "I didn't waste any time. I made an appointment with my ophthalmologist right away."

The examination showed that Paul's vision had declined to 6/21 (20/70) in his left eye. "The ophthalmologist told me that my visual acuity did not permit me to drive anymore, as it no longer met legal requirements," says Paul. "I was really disappointed to have to stop driving, as I had been a volunteer chauffeur for years," Paul explains. "I like being helpful and meeting people, and I was determined to do everything possible to find another activity that could meet my needs and get me out of the house."

Paul soon started a series of treatments involving monthly injections of ranibizumab (Lucentis®). Imagine his joy on realizing after several injections that his vision had improved considerably ... enough for him to be able to drive again! "I would never have believed it possible," says Paul. "I didn't even have time to find a new volunteer activity. Within a few months, I was able to return to my former activities, and the people I was chauffeuring were delighted to see me back on the road!"

CHAPTER 6
LIVING WITH AMD

A diagnosis of AMD is not a sentence to the life of a shut-in. Yes, the more advanced the stage of the disease, the greater the impact on your life and your ability to function. However, there are many optical, electronic and computerized aids as well as vision rehabilitation programs to help overcome physical and psychological difficulties and remain independent.

Services available in low vision rehabilitation centres provide an assessment of functional vision and help in developing independent reading, writing and getting around. In many cases, these services even make it possible for people with AMD to take courses, keep their jobs or find an accommodated job.

Most people are shocked to discover they have a visual impairment, but the vast majority learn to adapt.

LOW VISION REHABILITATION

When there is a major loss of central vision, the patient can enter a vision rehabilitation program in a specialized centre to learn how to use his or her remaining vision. In Canada, vision rehabilitation services are offered free of charge based on certain criteria (field of vision, visual acuity, etc.).

Eccentric viewing training

This program teaches how to use eccentric vision (vision outside the macula). This is essential for rehabilitating people with AMD, as it is directly related to activities of daily living, reading and writing. Instead of looking straight ahead, the person learns, through different exercises and tests, to use eccentric or peripheral vision. The preferred eccentric fixation point can be to the left or right, up or down, depending on the retinal lesions. Different exercises are used to determine which area of eccentric vision gives the clearest image.

The rehabilitation generally takes several months. However, it is impossible to say with any accuracy exactly how long it will take, as it depends on the severity of the AMD, the visual needs of the person and the speed of assimilation of the techniques taught. The training can sometimes cause fatigue or headaches, but it is important not to get discouraged.

By the end of the rehabilitation period, the person with AMD will have maximized his or her existing vision.

DON'T BE BLINDED BY LIGHT

People with AMD are easily blinded by sunlight or glare. Goggles, which offer lateral protection, are thus recommended. Some models have contrast enhancement filters. Recently manufacturers have been making an effort to improve the look of these goggles, and more and more models are available.

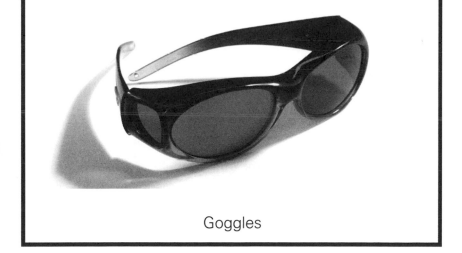

Goggles

VISION AIDS AND OTHER USEFUL PRODUCTS

Having a vision impairment or "low vision" does not mean you are blind. This means vision aids can be used to optimize remaining vision.

Some provinces have financial assistance programs for procurement of these assistive devices. Eligibility criteria include visual acuity and field of vision, income, benefit and retirement plans, age and occupational status. Vision aids can be loaned to eligible people or purchased from stores that specialize in adaptive products.

Optometrists (and sometimes ophthalmologists) recommend and prescribe vision aids based on the residual vision, capabilities and visual needs of the person with AMD. Some are used only for near vision, others are for far vision and still others are multifunctional. However, all require an adjustment and learning period.

Vision aids

Different optical systems use special lenses to enlarge the image for reading or writing.

Magnifiers

Magnifiers come in different shapes, strengths and sizes. Some have a built-in adjustable lighting system. There are handheld and pocket magnifiers, bar magnifiers and stand magnifiers (*Figure* ❶).

Electronic glasses

These lightweight, battery-operated glasses provide 50 times magnification up close and 30 times at a distance. They are used for theatre, cinema or television and can be converted to a standard magnifier for reading or writing. They transmit magnified, real-time, colour images of both near and far objects.

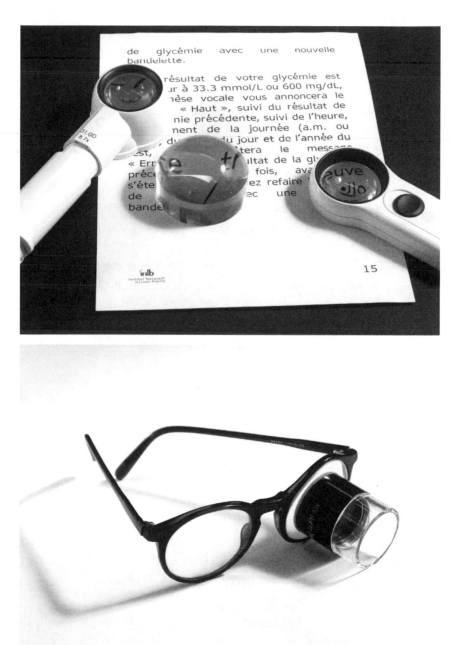

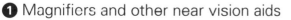

❶ Magnifiers and other near vision aids

Telescopes

A small telescope that can be clipped onto one or both lenses of a pair of glasses as needed can be used to improve distance vision. Recently, the U.S. Food and Drug Administration (FDA) approved a telescopic eye implant for certain cases of very advanced AMD. A telescope the size of a pencil eraser is implanted in the eye, replacing the eye's lens (*Figure* ❷).

Closed circuit televisions (CCTVs)

These devices use video technology to magnify letters to the desired size for reading and project them onto a screen. Contrast and brightness can be adjusted. CCTVs have a tray on which the book, magazine or document to be read is placed and a screen above it where the text is displayed in the character size selected by the user. CCTVs can also be used for writing (*Figure* ❸).

Computer applications

Different software makes it possible to read or write documents on a computer.

Screen readers

These programs convert printed documents (books, newspaper articles, etc.) that have been scanned into electronic documents that can be saved on a computer. The programs can even read electronic documents out loud, magnify the text on screen and modify the colour contrast to improve visibility.

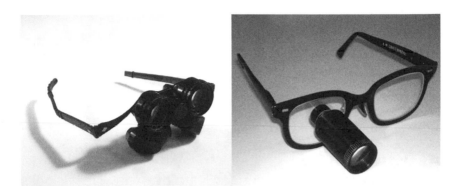

❷ Binocular and monocular telescopic systems

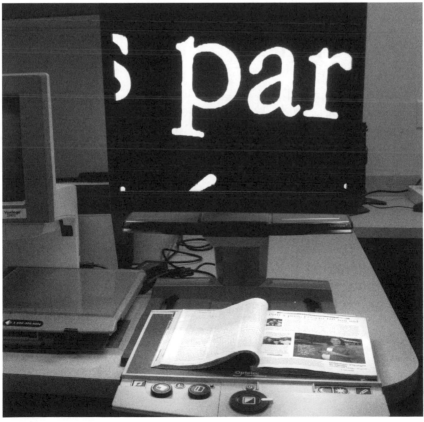

❸ Closed circuit television (CCTV)

Screen magnifiers

These programs magnify text, graphics and images displayed on a computer screen. Some screen magnifiers also magnify the mouse pointer and text cursor, and others allow the user to adjust the degree of magnification (*Figure* ❹).

Assistive devices

A variety of assistive devices facilitate everyday life—clocks with large numbers, big-button telephones, TV magnifying screens and talking thermostats, for example.

ADAPTING THE HOME

Certain home adaptations can improve the comfort and safety of people with AMD and help them stay in their own homes and remain independent. Sometimes it's just a question of adjusting the lighting to make the home functional, as people with AMD need more lighting to enhance contrasts.

The low vision rehabilitation specialist will rarely recommend that a person with AMD move, unless access to the home is unsafe (too many steps, for example).

The adaptation may consist of putting reflective strips on stair treads to mark the beginning and end of each step, making locks more accessible or using tactile stickers to mark the most commonly used temperatures on the stove.

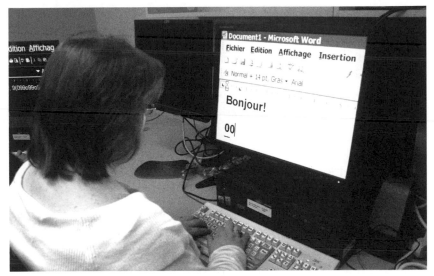

❹ Screen magnifier

ADAPTING THE WORKPLACE

A diagnosis of AMD does not necessarily mean losing your job. Employers are more and more open to the idea of adapting the workplace, when possible, to keep an employee. In Quebec, if you are eligible for the government assistance program, a low vision rehabilitation specialist will even meet with your employer to help assess your work station. Software to magnify text and images on a computer screen can also be borrowed. If you are unable to keep your job, you will be offered career counselling services and training programs to help you find a new job

GETTING AROUND

Anyone living with a visual impairment has special needs and varying degrees of difficulty getting around.

Even with low vision, travel is possible—alone or with assistance, on foot or by taxi, public transit or paratransit.

On foot

When visual impairment makes getting around on foot less safe or more difficult, a white cane or accompaniment is a solution. A white cane is not required with AMD, but some people feel more secure with a cane and use it to locate steps and obstacles. Others like to carry a white cane to alert strangers to their visual impairment.

Assistance from a friend or family member can be helpful when travelling to unknown places or in crowded areas.

Public transit

Many people with AMD use public transit daily. Subways are often more difficult than buses for people with severe visual impairments. The lighting is not the same from one station to the next, and accesses are totally different—with corridors and stairways of varying lengths. If the same route is taken regularly, it can be learned, so it becomes a familiar routine with known obstacles. An orientation and mobility specialist can help with this travel training.

Anyone with a visual acuity of 6/60 (20/200) or less, or a field of vision of 20 degrees or less, can obtain a CNIB ID card that entitles the holder to discounts on many public transit services.

Some non-profit organizations also provide transportation services with volunteer chauffeurs who drive their own cars. Last but not least, taxis or paratransit are good options when other ways of getting around seem complicated.

By car

Even with AMD, your vision may be good enough to drive a car. In Canada, visual acuity must be at least 6/15 (20/50) in the better eye to drive.

Sometimes the ophthalmologist or optometrist will ask a patient to hand over his or her driver's license. However, if the patient's vision improves enough with treatment, the license may be returned. Nonetheless, it is best to avoid driving at night, when there isn't much contrast and the risk of blinding by headlights is higher. Paratransit services are offered in most parts of Canada.

HELP FROM FAMILY

AMD can have a major psychological impact. It affects not only your mobility and independence but also your self-image. Support from close friends and family members is crucial. Friends and family, who are often very upset by the diagnosis, can receive advice and explanations during a visit to the optometrist or ophthalmologist, or a meeting with a rehabilitation specialist.

The friends and family of a person with AMD are also the first to want to help with daily living activities. However, they may tend to do things for you, especially if they don't know what you can do by yourself. It's best if they offer help, which you can refuse if not needed, instead of just doing things for you.

The reactions of friends and family are crucial for the person with AMD. They can affect your self-esteem and rehabilitation. If you feel that your family does not accept your condition, you will have difficulty accepting it yourself and making the necessary efforts to remain independent. Worse yet, certain reactions can affect your feelings of self-worth and lead to depression. This is why it is so important that family and friends support and encourage the person with AMD.

SPECIALIZED PSYCHOSOCIAL SERVICES

The emotional aspect of vision loss is one of the biggest difficulties to overcome. When you learn you have AMD, you may experience many emotions—shock, denial, anger, rage, sadness. These may occur in any order and with any intensity, and may last for any length of time. Some people relive the different stages of grief with every vision change, even when they are prepared and have been through it before.

A person with AMD may even go through a period of depression, in which case help must be found. Support groups and organizations that provide psychological assistance are available for people with AMD (*see Useful Addresses*). Your eye specialist will even refer you to a psychologist if you feel the need. However, the services offered in a low vision rehabilitation centre, together with monitoring by an ophthalmologist, are often enough to dispel worries and fears and move past the initial state of shock. One thing is certain: accepting the disease helps the person with AMD to adjust to the changes and remain confident and independent.

ONE PERSON'S STORY

Name: Sylvia	Age: 58
Occupation: Teacher	

Sylvia was a teacher in an elementary school when she learned at age 58 that she had wet AMD. "My husband and children were very reassuring and helped me a great deal in accepting the diagnosis. At home I had my points of reference and could count on my family to help me when I really needed them. At school, however, it was a different story," she says.

Sylvia was not yet old enough to retire and wanted to teach for a few more years, but her poor visual acuity made her work more difficult. "In the first months following my diagnosis, I wasn't willing to change any of my habits or teaching methods. I refused to work with visual aids ... until the day I understood that was how I would keep my job," she confides. Her students were thus informed of her disease, and a professional from the low vision rehabilitation centre even came to her class to show them the magnifier and closed circuit television she would be using every day.

Thanks to these visual aids, Sylvia was able to continue teaching until her retirement. "I was worried for so long about the reaction of my students, but in the end I was pleasantly surprised by their behaviour. To my great astonishment, they were less rowdy and more attentive when I read to them using the closed circuit television," she explains. "They would even bring me my magnifier when I would forget it on a student's desk as I moved around the classroom."

CHAPTER 7
TREATMENTS OF
THE FUTURE

AMD research is very active at present and has substantial financial support. Advances are being made rapidly, giving hope that future treatments will be even more effective in limiting complications and repairing lesions—and that prevention may even be possible. With the extraordinary progress in research on new therapies, no one can predict today how AMD will be treated ten or even five years from now. We are witnessing an explosion in research which is generating much hope. Though results are expected in the medium rather than the short term, the future looks promising.

FUTURE DRUGS

In the years ahead, new drugs now being studied may offer treatment for people with dry AMD. We know little at the moment about these new treatments being developed by pharmaceutical companies. We do know, however, that the research is advancing, as a number of studies with human subjects have already been conducted. For example, antiinflammatories are being developed to counter the key role played by inflammation in the progression and probably even the onset of dry AMD.

These new drugs will probably be administered as drops.

FUTURE ANTIANGIOGENIC THERAPIES

Current research is directed mainly at improving existing treatments for wet AMD. Doctors now have medications that can be injected into the vitreous humour of the eye. These antiangiogenic (or anti-VEGF) therapies cause lesions to stabilize and even regress. However, the injections have to be repeated every four to six weeks. Researchers are keenly interested in developing sustained-release delivery systems so antiangiogenics can act continuously. One option being studied is implantation of biodegradable capsules containing extended-release antiangiogenic agents in the vitreous body.

A number of anti-VEGFs are currently under development— including VEGF-Trap (prevents VEGF from binding to its receptors) and SiRNA (suppresses VEGF production). The goal is to develop new and more effective ways to prevent neovascularization or to directly attack VEGF, the protein responsible for inducing neovascularization.

GENE THERAPY

Several AMD-related genes have been discovered recently. We know, as a result, that AMD is associated not with a single gene but a genetic constellation—complicating the research. These genetic discoveries have nonetheless provided new insight into the disease and suggested new treatment and prevention avenues, including gene therapy.

Gene therapy consists in altering the genetic make-up of the cells involved in AMD to prevent onset of the disease. The idea is to alter the structure of the defective gene in the cell so it will fight the disease. A viral vector will be used to introduce a suitable genetic code. The virus used will have the ability to penetrate the cell and insert its DNA in the host nucleus and chromosomes. The patient's cells can then produce the proteins that fight or correct the AMD. The main challenge in this therapeutic approach is to prevent disease progression by targeting the molecules involved.

Gene therapy is a future treatment for prevention of AMD. Additional studies are required to develop clinical applications. Though still in the experimental stage, genetic therapies may nonetheless become available for people with AMD in the years ahead. In the longer term, when we have a better understanding of the genes that predispose to AMD, genetic therapy will probably be considered as preventive treatment.

STEM CELL TRANSPLANTATION

Retinal transplants are not a conceivable option at the moment for people with AMD. However, scientists do hope to one day be able to repair retinal damage caused by AMD by producing retinal cells and transplanting them in the eye. These cells would then multiply to replace those that have disappeared. Some researchers thus believe that stem cell transplantation will restore vision in people with AMD. Transplantation of stem cells genetically modified to produces genes that protect against progression of AMD is another possibility.

These procedures, however, involve very long-term research. We do not expect to be transplanting stem cells in the near future, as there are still technical problems. Though these techniques are not foreseeable in the short term, there is nonetheless reason for much hope.

USEFUL ADDRESSES

CANADA

AMD Alliance International
1929 Bayview Avenue
Toronto, Ontario M4G 3E8
1-416-486-2500 or 1-877-AMD-7171
www.amdalliance.org

Organization offering information and assistance for people with AMD and their families.

Audible.com
www.audible.com
Over 75,000 audiobooks available for download for a fee.

Canadian Association of Optometrists (CAO)
234 Argyle Avenue
Ottawa, Ontario K2P 1B9
1-888-263-4676
www.opto.ca

The professional association of optometrists in Canada. It is also the national federation of 10 provincial associations of optometrists.

Canadian Ophthalmological Society
610-1525 Carling Avenue
Ottawa, Ontario K1Z 8R9
1-613-729-6779
www.eyesite.ca

Canadian association of physicians and surgeons specializing in eye care.

CNIB
1929 Bayview Avenue
Toronto, Ontario M4G 3E8
1-800-563-2642
www.inca.ca

Nationwide, community-based, registered charity committed to research, public education and vision health for all Canadians.

CNIB Library
1929 Bayview Avenue Toronto, ON M4G 3E8
1-800-563-2642
http://www.cnib.ca/en/services/library

Offers access to thousands of titles in braille and printbraille as well as audio books, newspapers and magazine, descriptive videos and document search services. Alternate-media books and other documents can be consulted online or delivered on loan postage-free.

VoicePrint
1-800-567-6755
www.voiceprintcanada.com

A 24-hour reading service operated by The National Broadcast Reading Service. VoicePrint broadcasts readings of full-text articles 24/7 from more than 600 Canadian newspapers and magazines.

QUEBEC

Association québécoise de la dégénérescence maculaire
C.P. 47595, COP Plateau Mont-Royal
Montréal (QC) H2H 1S8
450-651-5747 or 1-866-867-9389
www.degenerescencemaculaire.ca

This association directs people with AMD to existing medical, technological and sociocultural resources and provides information on prevention, treatments and research conducted around the world.

Association des médecins ophtalmologistes du Québec
2, Complexe Desjardins
C.P. 216, succursale Desjardins
Montréal (QC) H5B 1G8
514-350-5124
www.amoq.org

Quebec association of ophthalmologists. The Web site provides information on AMD.

Association des optométristes du Québec
1265, rue Berri, bureau 740
Montréal (QC) H2L 4X4
514-288-6272
www.aoqnet.qc.ca

Quebec association of optometrists. The Web site provides information for the public.

Audiothèque
4765, 1re Avenue, bureau 210
Québec (QC) G1H 2T3
1-877-393-0103
www.audiotheque.net/

Information centre for people without access to written materials. Users have telephone access to readings of newspaper articles, magazines, circulars and any other written material.

Centre de réadaptation, d'orientation et d'intégration au travail
750, boulevard Marcel-Laurin, bureau 450
Saint-Laurent (QC) H4M 2M4
514-744-2944
www.aimcroitqc.org/aproposdenous.htm

Accommodated job search assistance for people with visual impairments and workplace adaptation assistance for employers.

Comité d'adaptation de la main-d'œuvre pour personnes handicapées (CAMO)

55, avenue du Mont-Royal Ouest
Bureau 300, 3ᵉ étage
Montréal (QC) H2T 2S6
514-522-3310 or 1-888-522-3310
www.camo.qc.ca/

Provincial committee whose mission is to promote access to training and employment for people living with handicaps.

Institut Nazareth et Louis-Braille

1111, rue Saint-Charles Ouest
Longueuil (QC) J4K 5G4
450-463-1710 or 1-800-361-7063
www.inlb.qc.ca

Low vision rehabilitation centre providing services for people with total or partial vision loss.

L'Institut de réadaptation en déficience physique de Québec (IRDPQ)

525, boulevard Wilfrid-Hamel
Québec (QC) G1M 2S8
418-529-9141
www.irdpq.qc.ca/

Offers a rehabilitation program for people with visual impairments and access to optical aids to compensate for visual loss.

La Magnétothèque

1055, boulevard René-Lévesque Est, bureau 501
Montréal (QC) H2L 4S5
1-800-361-0635
www.lamagnetotheque.qc.ca/

Close to 10,000 audio books: novels, philosophy, psychology, biographies, etc. Volunteers also read editorials and articles from Quebec newspapers.

Service québécois du livre adapté (SQLA)

475, boulevard De Maisonneuve Est
Montréal (QC) H2L 5C4
514-873-4454 or 1-866-410-0844
www.banq.qc.ca/portal/dt/sqla/sqla.htm

A French-language adapted book collection (Braille and audio books) available at the Grande Bibliothèque.

UNITED STATES

American Macular Degeneration Foundation

P.O. Box 515
Northampton, MA 01061-0515
1 413-268-7660
www.macular.org

Association for Macular Diseases
210 East 64th Street, 8th Floor
New York, NY 10065
1-212-605-3719
www.macula.org

The Macular Degeneration Foundation
P.O. Box 531313
Henderson, Nevada 89053
1-702-450-2908
www.eyesight.org

Macular Degeneration International
1-800-683-5555
www.maculardegeneration.org

The Macular Degeneration Partnership
6222 Wilshire Blvd., Suite 260
Los Angeles, CA 90048
1-310-623-4466
www.amd.org

Macular Degeneration Support
3600 Blue Ridge Blvd.
Grandview, MO 64030
1-816-761-7080
www.mdsupport.org

GLOSSARY

Amsler grid: a grid formed of horizontal and vertical lines (generally white lines on a black ground) and used to detect distortions of images perceived in the central visual field (metamorphopsia).

Antioxidants: substances that help protect the cells of the body against harmful waste (free radicals) produced by the body or from outside sources (chemicals, dust, etc.). Common antioxidants include vitamin C, vitamin E, selenium and the carotenoids (beta carotene, lycopene and lutein).

Anti-VEGF: medication that suppresses the growth of abnormal blood vessels (neovascularization) and reduces their permeability.

Atrophic AMD: loss of vision cells and retinal pigment epithelium cells. Also called geographic atrophy.

Autofluorescence: the fluorescent property of certain substances, such as lipofuscin, in response to an exciting light.

Cataract: transformation of the lens of the eye, which gradually loses its natural transparency. This is called opacification and may be caused by age or disease.

Central vision: central part of the field of vision, responsible for high-resolution vision.

Classic neovascularization: neovascularization which is well-defined in fluorescein angiography.

Cone: cell responsible for fine-detail and colour vision.

Conjunctiva: membrane that lines the inside of the eyelid and covers the entire eyeball, except the cornea.

DNA: deoxyribonucleic acid, a molecule found in all living cells that contains all the information necessary for the development and functioning of an organism. It is also the genetic blueprint, because it is transmitted, in whole or in part, during reproduction. It thus carries the organism's genetic information and composes its genome.

Drusen: white spots that can be seen in an examination of the back of the eye (fundus examination). Drusen are waste material that the retina is unable to clear away.

Fluorescein angiography: an examination in which dye (fluorescein) is injected intravenously and the internal structures of the eye are then photographed.

Fovea: the centre of the macula, the region of the retina where fine-detail vision is sharpest.

Fundus examination: an examination of the back of the eye, namely the retina and the retinal blood vessels.

Genetic therapy: method of introducing genetic material (genes) into the cells of an organism to correct anomalies causing disease.

Indocyanine green angiography: an examination in which dye (indocyanine green) is injected intravenously and the internal structures of the eye are then photographed.

Intravitreal injection: a direct injection into the eye, through the white of the eye and into the vitreous cavity behind the lens.

Laser: a device for amplifying light and producing a narrow "coherent" beam of light. Different types of lasers are used in ophthalmology.

Legally blind: having a visual acuity of 6/20 (20/200) or less.

Lipofuscin: cellular pigment consisting of molecular debris naturally present in the back of the eye.

Macula: the central part of the retina.

Metamorphopsia: distortion of straight lines.

Neovascularization: growth of new, abnormal blood vessels.

Occult neovascularization: neovascularization which is poorly defined in fluorescein angiography.

Omega-3: polyunsaturated fatty acids found in large quantities in certain fatty fish as well as in nuts and canola oil.

Ophthalmologist: a medical doctor who specializes in diseases of the eye and related structures.

Optical coherence tomography (OCT): a scanning technology used to generate cross-sectional images of the retina, from the outermost to the deepest layers.

Optician: a person who sells optical instruments, including eyeglasses.

Optometrist: a vision professional who is not a medical doctor but is trained to diagnose and treat vision problems (with eyeglasses, contact lenses and eye exercises) and certain other eye health issues.

Peripheral vision: the outer part of the field of vision, controlled by rods.

Photodynamic therapy (PDT): a method of treatment involving low-energy laser irradiation after intravenous injection of a light-activated agent that will interact with the laser beam.

Rods: cells responsible for detecting motion in our field of vision and for night vision.

Snellen scale (or chart): standard scale used to measure visual acuity consisting of a chart with letters of progressively smaller size. Normal vision is 20/20 in feet or 6/6 in metres, which means a person with normal visual acuity can see all the letters on the chart from a distance of 20 feet or 6 metres.

Trace elements: iodine, copper, fluorine, chlorine, zinc, cobalt, selenium and manganese.

Ultrasound: a method of exploring the eye by measuring reflected echoes.

Vision aid: an optical system (magnifier, closed circuit television, etc.) used to magnify the retinal image with the help of special lenses. Also called an optical aid.

Vision rehabilitation: all of the techniques used to help a patient maximize the use of his or her remaining vision.

Visual acuity: the eye's capacity to recognize fine detail. The vision specialist uses the Snellen scale to measure visual acuity.